AGELESS YOGA

A Chair Yoga Guide for Seniors
60 and Beyond

Lizzy D. White

Copyright © 2023 by Lizzy D. White

Without the publisher's written consent, no portion of this book may be duplicated in any way, whether it be electronically or mechanically, including photocopying, recording, or by any information storage and retrieval system.

The information contained in this handbook is provided "as is" without any express or implied warranty of any kind. The authors, editors, and publishers of this work make no representations or warranties as to the accuracy or completeness of any information contained herein and disclaim any liability for any errors or omissions. The only goals of this work are informative and instructional. It isn't meant to take the place of expert medical guidance, diagnosis, or care. If you have any concerns about a medical problem, always seek the counsel of your doctor or another skilled healthcare professional. Never postpone getting professional medical care due to something you have read in this book, and never reject expert medical advice.

This book is not intended for use by children under the age of 18. Chair Yoga Guide for Seniors 60 and Beyond does not recommend or endorse any specific tests, physicians, products, procedures, or opinions mentioned in this book. You entirely assume all risk if you rely on any of the information given here. The trademarks, service marks, logos, and trade names used in this book are the property of their respective owners and are used for identification purposes only. This book is protected by copyright laws and treaties. Unauthorized reproduction or distribution of this book, or any portion of it, may result in severe civil and criminal penalties and will be prosecuted to the maximum extent possible under the law.

TABLE OF CONTENT

INTRODUCTION

CHAPTER ONE

THE BENEFITS OF YOGA FOR SENIOR HEALTH

The Importance of chair Yoga for Seniors

Chair Yoga: A safe and accessible practice

Understanding Senior Health

Common Health concerns and how Yoga can help

Importance of Balance and Mobility

CHAPTER TWO

SETTING UP YOUR YOGA SPACE

Choosing the Right Chair and Props

CHAPTER THREE

BASIC CHAIR YOGA POSES

Yoga for

CHAPTER FOUR

BREATHWORK AND MEDITATION

Yoga for Sleep

Yoga for Managing Chronic Pain

Creating a Sustainable Practice

Tips for Staying Consistent

CONCLUSION

INTRODUCTION

As a yogi, I had the privilege to introduce my elderly grandparents to chair yoga. At first, they were hesitant to try something new and unfamiliar, but after I took the time to explain the benefits of chair yoga, they were both eager to give it a try. My grandparent's first experience with chair yoga was incredibly rewarding. They found it to be an enjoyable and relaxing way to exercise with minimal impact on the joints and muscles.

After a few sessions, they reported feeling more energized, flexible, and mobile. Chair yoga is an excellent form of exercise for seniors, as it is both gentle and effective. Not only does chair yoga help to reduce pain and stiffness, but it can also improve balance, flexibility, posture, and circulation. Additionally, chair yoga is a great way for seniors to stay active and engaged, allowing them to maintain a higher quality of life. My grandparents are now regular practitioners of chair yoga and have seen tremendous improvements in their physical and mental well-being.

It has been a wonderful experience to witness the positive transformation in their health and well-being that chair yoga has brought about. If you are looking for an easy and effective exercise to improve your health and well-being, I highly recommend trying chair yoga for seniors. With so many benefits, it is an excellent way to stay active and healthy in your golden years.

Chair yoga is a great way for seniors to maintain an active lifestyle and experience the many benefits of yoga. It is a form of yoga that is specifically designed to be practiced while seated in a chair or while standing with the support of a chair. This makes it an ideal form of exercise for seniors with limited mobility or those who are looking for a gentle way to exercise. Chair yoga is beneficial for seniors in many ways.

It helps to reduce pain and stiffness, improve balance, flexibility, and posture, as well as enhance circulation. It is also a great way to reduce stress and anxiety, promote mental clarity, and improve overall well-being. My elderly grandparents are a testament to the positive effects of chair yoga. They have experienced a remarkable transformation in their physical and mental health since they began practicing chair yoga, they are now full of energy and enthusiasm.

If you are a senior looking for an easy and effective way to stay active and healthy, I highly recommend trying chair yoga. Chair yoga combines traditional yoga poses with the support of a chair to provide balance and stability. Chair yoga is a great way for seniors to get the physical and mental benefits of yoga without having to get up or down from the floor. With the help of a chair, seniors can modify poses to their comfort and ability level. Chair yoga is an excellent choice for seniors who want to stay active, improve their overall health and active lifestyle.

Chair yoga is a safe and gentle practice that is accessible to people of all ages and fitness levels, making it a great choice for seniors who want to stay active and improve their overall health.

CHAPTER ONE

THE BENEFITS OF YOGA FOR SENIOR HEALTH

Yoga is a great activity for seniors to maintain and improve their overall health and well-being. It is a form of exercise that is low-impact, gentle, and easy to modify to fit individual needs and abilities. Yoga can provide many benefits to seniors, including increased flexibility, strength, balance, and mental clarity. Flexibility As we age, it is common to experience stiffness and loss of flexibility. Yoga can help to improve flexibility, increase range of motion, and reduce joint discomfort.

Practicing yoga can help seniors stay fit and active, as well as improve their overall health. Physical Benefits Yoga is an excellent way for seniors to stay fit and active. It increases flexibility, strength, and balance, which can help prevent falls and other injuries common to older adults. Yoga can also help seniors improve their posture and build strength in their core muscles.

Mental Benefits Yoga can be a great way to reduce stress and improve mental clarity. It can also help seniors increase their focus and concentration, and help them stay in tune with their bodies. Yoga also encourages seniors to be in the present moment, allowing them to relax and appreciate the simple things in life. Improved Quality of Life Yoga can help seniors stay fit and active, as well as improve their overall quality of life. It can help them stay connected to their community, reduce anxiety, and improve their overall sense of well-being. Yoga is a great way for seniors to stay physically and mentally active. It can help them stay in shape and reduce the risk of injury, while also providing mental and emotional benefits.

The Importance of chair Yoga for Seniors

Chair yoga is a great way for seniors to stay fit and active while avoiding physical strain. Chair yoga is a form of yoga that is practiced while sitting in a chair, or while using the chair for support. It is designed to help seniors maintain their flexibility, strength, balance, and overall wellness. For seniors, chair yoga offers a variety of benefits. It can help reduce aches and pains, improve range of motion, and increase muscle strength and tone.

Chair yoga poses are designed to be gentle and low-impact, making them ideal for seniors who have limited mobility or who may be at risk of falling. Many of the poses can be done seated in a chair and can be modified for those who need more support. Chair yoga can also be done with a partner if needed. Chair yoga is an excellent way for seniors to stay fit, healthy, and connected with the world around them.

Chair Yoga: A safe and accessible practice

Understanding Senior Health

Senior health is an important topic to consider. As our population ages, we need to be aware of the health needs of the elderly and how best to meet them. Good senior health begins with regular checkups. Regular visits to the doctor can help identify potential health issues before they become serious.

These visits are even more important as we age, as our bodies become more vulnerable to disease and injury. Exercise is also important for senior health. Regular physical activity can help to keep seniors strong and active. It can also help to reduce the risk of falls, which can be a common problem for the elderly. Walking, swimming, yoga, and tai chi are all good forms of exercise for seniors.

Also, staying socially active is important for seniors health. Seniors should make an effort to stay in touch with family and friends, and to get involved in activities that interest them. This can help to reduce feelings of loneliness and depression, which can be common among seniors.

Chair yoga is an increasingly popular form of yoga that has become a favorite among seniors and those with disabilities or limited mobility. It is a low-impact form of exercise that can be done while seated in a chair, making it accessible to people of all ages and abilities. Chair yoga provides many of the same health benefits as traditional yoga, such as increased flexibility, improved strength, and better balance, while providing a safe and comfortable environment for seniors to practice.

It is also a great way to build strength, endurance, and coordination, and can be done at any fitness level. Chair yoga can be done in a group setting or individually, and requires minimal equipment. Chair yoga is also beneficial to seniors in terms of mental health. Studies have shown that practicing yoga can reduce symptoms of depression, anxiety, and stress. The practice of yoga can also help improve cognitive function and memory and can be a great way for seniors to socialize and stay connected with their peers. For seniors, chair yoga can be a great way to stay fit and healthy. It is low-impact, accessible to all levels of fitness, and can be done from the comfort of a chair.

Common Health concerns and how Yoga can help

Importance of Balance and Mobility

Yoga is an ancient exercise system that can be beneficial for people of all ages, including seniors. Balance and mobility are two important components of yoga for seniors, as they can help to improve physical health, reduce the risk of falls, and improve mental and emotional well-being.

Balance is essential for seniors, as it helps to maintain their independence and quality of life. Balance exercises, such as tree pose and warrior pose, can help to improve coordination and stability, allowing seniors to remain active and engaged in their daily activities. Balance exercises can also help to improve posture, reduce the risk of falls, and strengthen the legs and core.

Mobility is also important for seniors, as it helps to improve flexibility, range of motion, and strength. Mobility exercises, such as sun salutations and chair poses, can help to improve joint movement and reduce the risk of injury. Mobility exercises can also help to improve posture and help seniors move with ease and confidence. Yoga is a great way for seniors to improve their balance and mobility. It is a low-impact exercise that can be modified to suit any fitness level. It also helps to improve mental and emotional well-being, as it is a calming and meditative exercise.

In summary, balance and mobility are important components of yoga for seniors. Balance exercises can help to improve coordination and stability, while mobility exercises can help to improve flexibility and range of motion. Practicing yoga can help seniors remain independent and active.

CHAPTER TWO

SETTING UP YOUR YOGA SPACE

To make the most of their yoga practice, seniors should consider setting up their yoga space to accommodate their changing physical needs. When setting up a yoga space for seniors, consider the following:

1. **Use a supportive surface**: For comfort and safety, it's important to provide a supportive surface that won't slip or slide. A yoga mat or non-slip rug is ideal, as it will provide cushioning and grip. For those with limited mobility or balance, a

wall-mounted yoga strap or non-slip chair can provide additional stability.

2. **Provide adequate lighting**: Good lighting is essential for seniors, as it can help with balance and visibility. Place lamps around the yoga space to provide adequate lighting, and ensure that all lamps are positioned at a comfortable height for the individual.

3. **Consider the size and layout of the space**: Make sure that the yoga space is large enough to accommodate the senior's needs, and also consider the layout of the space. If the senior is using a wheelchair, it's important to ensure that there is enough space to move freely.

4. **Choose a comfortable temperature:** For seniors, a

comfortable temperature is critical. Consider installing a fan or air conditioning unit in the yoga space.

5. **Choose appropriate props**: Props such as blocks, straps, chairs, and bolsters can be beneficial for seniors, as they can help them to get into and hold poses more easily. Choose props that are comfortable and easy to use.

6. **Play calming music**: Music can be a great way to create a calming environment for yoga practice. Choose calming music that won't be too distracting.

7. **Make use of aromatherapy**: Aromatherapy can help to create a calming environment, and can also provide physical and emotional

benefits. Consider using essential oils or scented candles in the yoga space.

8. **Consider the visuals**: Visuals such as pictures and decorations can be used to create the right atmosphere for yoga practice. Choose calming visuals that the senior can enjoy.

9. **Set aside time for the practice**: To get the most out of the practice, it's important to set aside time for it. Make sure to schedule regular yoga sessions so that the senior can stay consistent.

10. **Check in with a doctor**: Before beginning a yoga practice, it's important to check in with a doctor to ensure that it's safe for the senior to do so.

Choosing the Right Chair and Props

To make the most of this type of yoga, it is important to choose the right chair and props for the practice. Here are some tips on how to select the best chair and props for chair yoga for seniors:

1. **Choose a chair with a comfortable seat.** Chair yoga for seniors should be done in a chair with a comfortable cushion and good back and arm support. Look for an adjustable chair, so that it can fit your senior's body type and height. Consider the weight capacity of the chair, as seniors may have limited mobility and strength.
2. **Look for a chair with a stable base.** Chair yoga for seniors should be

done in a chair that is stable and won't be easily moved. Make sure the chair has a wide base that is well-balanced and can support the senior's weight.

3. **Choose proper props**. To make chair yoga more effective, certain props may be necessary. Look for props that are lightweight and easy to transport. Consider getting props that can be attached to the chair, such as straps or handles, so that seniors can easily grip them while doing the exercises.

4. **Consider the environment**. Chair yoga for seniors should be done in a safe, comfortable environment. Make sure the chair is placed on a flat, stable surface and away from any potential

hazards. Look for a space that is well-lit and has good ventilation.

With the right chairs, supportive floor surface, clear instructions, and a peaceful atmosphere, seniors can enjoy the physical, mental and emotional benefits of chair yoga in a safe and comfortable environment.

CHAPTER THREE

BASIC CHAIR YOGA POSES

Mountain Pose: Mountain Pose is a seated pose that helps to improve posture, balance, and circulation. The pose strengthens the spine, hips, and legs while calming the mind. Seniors need to practice this pose to ensure their bodies maintain strong and healthy postures. This pose starts with the feet together and arms at the side. The body is upright with the head and neck in line with the spine. The torso is in a neutral position, chest open and shoulders relaxed. As the pose is held, the practitioner focuses on the breath and lengthening the spine.

Chair Warrior: Chair Warrior is a seated chair pose that strengthens the legs, arms, and core while improving balance. It also increases the range of motion and flexibility. This pose is beneficial for seniors to practice as it helps maintain strength and balance and can help prevent falls. This pose begins in a seated position on the chair. The feet are firmly placed on the floor and the hands are placed on the armrests of the chair. The practitioner then inhales, and as they exhale, they lean forward, keeping the spine straight and reaching the arms forward. The head looks slightly forward and the gaze is focused on the hands.

Seated Sun Salutation: Seated Sun Salutation is a series of seated poses that focus on stretching the body and calming the mind. It increases circulation, strengthens the muscles, and improves flexibility. This pose is important for seniors to practice as it can help reduce stress and improve their overall well-being. This pose starts in a seated position, with the feet together and arms at the sides. As the practitioner inhales, they raise their arms above the head and arch their back, creating an arch in the spine. As they exhale, they bring their arms back to the sides, and then fold forward, keeping the spine straight and the head nodding towards the chest.

Cat-Cow: Cat-Cow is a seated pose that helps to improve balance, flexibility, and posture while calming the mind. It helps to stretch the spine and neck while strengthening the arms and legs. This pose is important to practice for seniors as it can help to reduce stiffness and improve range of motion. This pose starts on hands and knees with the wrists directly below the shoulders and the knees directly below the hips. As the practitioner inhales, they arch the spine and tilt the head up, looking towards the ceiling. As they exhale, they round the spine, tucking the chin towards the chest and stretching the neck downwards.

Intermediate Chair Yoga Poses: Intermediate Chair Yoga Poses are more challenging poses for seniors that focus on increasing balance, flexibility, and strength.

These poses can help to improve the range of motion and can also reduce stiffness. Seniors need to practice these poses to ensure their bodies stay strong and healthy.

This pose starts in a seated position on the chair. The feet are firmly placed on the floor and the arms are extended outward. The practitioner then inhales and as they exhale, they lean forward, keeping the spine straight and reaching the arms forward. The head looks slightly forward and the gaze is focused on the hands. The practitioner then inhales and as they exhale, they bring the arms back to the body, leaning back and arching the spine. The head looks slightly upward and the gaze is focused on the ceiling

Chair Triangle: This pose is done while seated in a chair. Place your feet hip-width apart and reach your right arm up to the sky, then bend over to the left, reaching your right arm towards the floor and your left arm towards the ceiling. Before swapping sides, hold for a few breaths. This pose helps to improve flexibility in the spine and shoulders and can help to reduce pain and stiffness in these areas.

Seated Twist: Start with your feet flat on the floor and your hands resting on your knees. Inhale deeply and as you exhale, twist your upper body to the right and place your left hand on the back of the chair. Hold for several breaths, then switch sides. This pose helps to improve circulation and digestion, as well as relieve tension in the spine and back.

Extended Side Angle: Begin in a seated position with your feet flat on the floor. Reach your right arm up to the sky and then exhale as you bring your right arm down and out to the side. Bend your right knee and rest your right arm along the outside of your right leg. Before swapping sides, hold for a few breaths. This pose helps to improve flexibility in the hips and spine, as well as strengthen the abdominal muscles.

Chair Downward-Facing Dog is a gentle, restorative pose that helps to improve balance and flexibility. This pose can also be used to help seniors reduce stress and tension. In this pose, the senior sits on the edge of their chair with their feet flat on the floor. Then, they slowly lower their torso towards the floor, allowing their arms to relax and reach toward the ground. This pose will help to strengthen the spine, improve circulation, and increase joint flexibility. It will also help to reduce stiffness in the back and hips.

Chair Handstand: This pose is great for improving balance and strengthening the core muscles. It is important for seniors as it helps with maintaining balance, which can be particularly important as they age. This pose is done by sitting on the edge of a chair, feet flat on the ground, and then lifting the feet off the ground. The hands should be placed firmly on the seat of the chair for balance.

Headstand Preparation: This pose is a great way for seniors to improve their strength and balance. Seniors need to practice this pose because it helps to strengthen the core muscles, which can be beneficial for preventing falls. This pose is done by sitting on the edge of a chair with the feet flat on the ground. The arms should be placed on the seat of the chair and used to lift the legs until they are perpendicular to the floor.

Shoulder Stand: This pose is an important one for seniors because it helps to improve posture and balance. It is done by sitting on the edge of a chair with the feet flat on the ground. The arms should be used to lift the legs until they are perpendicular to the floor. The arms should then be used to support the body as the legs are slowly lowered down until the back and shoulders are resting on the ground.

Plow Pose: This pose is beneficial for seniors because it helps to increase flexibility and improve posture. It is done by sitting on the edge of a chair with the feet flat on the ground. The arms should be used to lift the legs until they are perpendicular to the floor. The arms should then be used to support the body as the legs are slowly lowered down until the back and shoulders are resting on the ground. The legs should then be slowly raised overhead until the toes are pointing to the ceiling. Yoga for Specific

Standing Balance Poses: This pose helps to improve balance and posture by engaging and strengthening the core muscles. Gentle Chair Flow: This pose helps to improve flexibility, circulation, and range of motion while also providing a gentle and calming effect.

Seated Strengthening Poses: This pose helps to improve strength and posture by engaging and strengthening the core muscles.

Health Concerns: This type of yoga is great for seniors as it can be tailored to their specific needs. This type of yoga can help with issues such as arthritis, joint pain, and other age-related health concerns. Seniors need to practice this type of yoga because it is gentle and can be adapted to each individual's needs.

Yoga for

Yoga for Arthritis: This pose helps to reduce pain and stiffness associated with arthritis. Additionally, the joints' suppleness and range of motion are enhanced.

Yoga for Osteoporosis: This pose helps to improve bone density and strength, which is especially beneficial for those with osteoporosis. Additionally, the joints' suppleness and range of motion are enhanced.

Yoga for Heart Health: This pose helps to improve heart health by increasing circulation, breathing deeply, and reducing stress.

Yoga for Stress Management and Relaxation: This pose helps to reduce stress and improve relaxation by focusing on the breath and releasing tension in the body.

CHAPTER FOUR

BREATHWORK AND MEDITATION

Breathwork and meditation are two powerful tools for managing stress, improving mental and physical health, and deepening your spiritual connection. When practiced together, breathwork and meditation can be a powerful combination for finding peace, clarity, and joy in your life. Breathwork is a practice that helps you increase your awareness of your breath and its effects on your body and mind. It involves consciously controlling your breathing rhythmically and mindfully. This can be done through a variety of different methods, such as pranayama, qigong, and yoga breathing exercises.

Breathwork can help to reduce stress, improve concentration, enhance creativity, and increase feelings of tranquility and connection. Meditation is a practice of focusing your awareness on the present moment. It can involve focusing on your breath, an object of meditation, or a mantra. Through meditation, you can develop a greater sense of inner peace, reduce stress, and cultivate an attitude of acceptance and appreciation. When practiced together, breathwork and meditation can help you to become more aware of your body and its needs, while also creating a sense of calm and clarity that can help to reduce stress and anxiety.

Additionally, the combination of breathwork and meditation can help to deepen your spiritual connection and can be an incredibly powerful tool for personal growth and transformation. If you're interested in trying out breathwork and meditation, start by choosing a comfortable place to practice and a time that works for you.

Make sure you are focused and avoid any form of distraction. Once you're comfortable, start by focusing your attention on your breath and letting it guide you. As you become more relaxed, you can begin to explore different breathwork techniques and meditation practices. With regular practice, you can experience the many benefits that breathwork and meditation can offer.

Yoga for Sleep

Yoga for Sleep for seniors is a great way to get a good night's rest without having to resort to prescription medications. As we age, our bodies become more sensitive to the effects of stress, and our sleep patterns can become disrupted. Yoga offers a gentle, non-invasive way to help promote restful sleep in seniors. Yoga can help reduce stress and anxiety that can interfere with sleep. Meditation and breathing exercises can help to clear the mind of negative thoughts and worries that can keep us awake at night. Certain postures can help to relax the body and provide a sense of calm. Yoga can also help to improve circulation, which can help to ensure that the body gets the oxygen it needs to function properly and promote a good night's rest. Certain poses can even help to reduce pain and discomfort that can keep seniors up at night.

Yoga can also help improve sleep, which can help reduce pain. It can help regulate breathing and can help relax the body and mind, which can help reduce stress and improve sleep quality.

Finally, yoga can help seniors to build strength and flexibility, which can help to improve posture, reduce fatigue, and promote better sleep. If you're a senior who is having trouble sleeping, why not give yoga a try? It's a safe and gentle way to promote restful sleep, and can even help to reduce stress and anxiety and improve overall health and well-being.

Yoga for Managing Chronic Pain

Yoga has become an increasingly popular form of exercise for seniors suffering from chronic pain. It can provide a range of benefits that can help ease pain and make daily activities easier. Yoga is a gentle form of exercise that can help strengthen and stretch muscles and joints, which can help reduce aches and pains.

It can also help improve posture and balance, which can increase mobility and decrease the risk of falls. Yoga can also help reduce stress and anxiety, which can help reduce pain. It can help increase the release of endorphins, the body's natural painkillers, which can help reduce pain. Yoga can also help improve flexibility, which can help reduce stiffness and improve the range of motion. This can help reduce pain and make daily activities easier. Yoga can also help build strength, which can help reduce pain and improve balance. It can also help improve mental clarity, which can help reduce pain.

Yoga is a safe form of exercise for seniors with chronic pain. It is important to find a yoga class that is designed specifically for seniors and that is taught by an experienced instructor. The instructor should be able to provide modifications to poses if needed and should be able to help ensure that the poses are done safely and correctly.

Incorporating Yoga into Your Daily Routine

Incorporating yoga into their daily routine can help them maintain their physical health, reduce stress and anxiety, and improve overall wellness. Physical Health Yoga provides a low-impact form of exercise that is gentle on the body. It can help seniors increase their range of motion, improve strength and balance, and reduce the risk of falls. Yoga can also help to relieve aches and pains associated with aging, such as arthritis and stiffness.

Mental Health Yoga can help to reduce stress and anxiety, as well as promote relaxation and mindfulness. Studies have shown that yoga can improve mental clarity and focus, as well as help reduce symptoms of depression. Practicing yoga can also help seniors to cultivate a sense of peace and well-being. Spiritual Health Yoga can be a powerful tool for connecting with the spiritual self. Through meditation, breathing exercises, and thoughtful movements, seniors can access a sense of inner peace and calm. Incorporating yoga into your daily routine is an excellent way for seniors to maintain their physical and mental health, as well as to connect with their spiritual selves. With regular practice, seniors can enjoy improved balance, strength, flexibility, and mental clarity.

Creating a Sustainable Practice

Creating a sustainable practice for seniors can be a challenging task. Seniors often require extra care and attention, and many of their needs differ from those of other age groups. To create a sustainable practice for seniors, healthcare professionals must take into account the special needs of this population, as well as the financial and other resources available to them.

1. It is important to understand the senior population and their needs. Seniors often have different health conditions than younger patients, and many have limited mobility and require assistance with everyday tasks. They may also be on a limited budget, so finding affordable care is essential.
2. Healthcare providers should create a comfortable environment and invite seniors. This can be done by providing a variety of activities that seniors can take part in, such as exercise classes,

social groups, and educational programs. Additionally, healthcare providers should consider installing equipment that is designed to meet the needs of seniors, such as adjustable exam tables and grab bars in bathrooms.

3. Healthcare providers should create systems that make it easy for seniors to access the care they need. This includes making sure that appointments and other necessary services are available promptly and that there are support services in place for seniors who need additional help. Healthcare providers should take into account the unique needs of seniors when selecting medical treatments and procedures.

4. Healthcare providers should strive to create a sustainable practice for seniors by making sure that they can maintain their financial stability. This can be done by working with insurance providers to ensure that seniors can access the care they need, as well as offering discounts and other incentives for seniors who need to stretch their budgets. healthcare providers should look for ways to reduce costs, such as utilizing telemedicine services. Creating a sustainable practice for seniors requires a special focus on their needs and the resources available to them. By understanding the special needs and challenges of the senior population, healthcare providers can

create a practice that is tailored to their needs and provides the care they need in a comfortable and inviting atmosphere.

Tips for Staying Consistent

Yoga is an incredibly beneficial form of exercise for seniors, as it helps to improve balance, flexibility, and overall strength. However, it can be difficult to stay consistent with a yoga practice. Here are some tips for staying consistent with your yoga practice as a senior:

1. **Set realistic goals**: Before you begin your yoga practice, it's important to set realistic goals for yourself. Consider how much time you can realistically commit to your practice,

and create a schedule that works for you.

2. **Start slowly**: When you're just starting, it's important to start slowly and focus on mastering the basics. As you progress, you can add more complex poses and flows to your practice.

3. **Find the right class**: It's important to find a class that is specifically designed for seniors. Many yoga studios offer classes specifically for seniors, or you can look for classes online.

4. **Make it a habit**: The key to staying consistent is to make it a habit. Try to practice at the same time each day or week and make it a part of your routine.

5. **Find a supportive community**: Find a supportive community that can help keep you motivated and inspired. Whether it's a group of friends or an online community, having a supportive group can help you stay consistent with your practice.

With dedication and commitment, you can reap the many benefits of yoga for seniors. continue to learn and enjoy your practice!

CONCLUSION

Congratulations on completing this course on yoga for seniors! You now have a better understanding of the different types of yoga, the health benefits of yoga, and how to safely practice yoga as a senior. We hope that the information and resources provided in this course have been helpful and have given you the confidence to continue your yoga journey. Resources There are many resources available to help you continue your yoga journey. Look for online yoga classes, local yoga studios, and even books and videos about yoga for seniors. You can also find helpful tips and advice from other seniors who practice yoga. Consider attending a yoga retreat or workshop to further your practice and deepen your understanding. With the right resources and guidance, you can continue to enjoy the physical, mental, and spiritual benefits of yoga.

Printed in the USA
CPSIA information can be obtained
at www.ICGtesting.com
CBHW072321230924
14838CB00008B/459